# All About
# SKIN CARE IN THE ELDERLY

By Lyla Reichart and V. M. Taylor, medical writers

The publisher would like to acknowledge the work of Laura Flynn R.N., B.N., M.B.A. as a major contributor to the concept of this book and the best practice guidelines from various authoritative organizations such as the WOCN (Wound Ostomy Continence Nurses) Association, the JCAHCO (Joint Commission on Accreditation of Home Care organizations), the RNAO (Royal Nurses Association of Ontario) and the CAWC (Canadian Association of Wound Care) and the NPUAB (National Pressure Ulcer Association Board).

Other contributors include the following nurse educators:

Wound care nurses, both ETs and WOCN members, who advised on the this project.

ISBN No: 978 1 896616 86 5

© 2013 Mediscript Communications Inc.

The publisher, Mediscript Communications Inc., acknowledges the financial support of the Government of Canada through the Canadian Book Fund for our publishing activities.

Printed in Canada

www.mediscript.net

Book and Front Cover design by:
Brian Adamson, www.AdamsonGraphics.net

SC1002011

# ALL ABOUT BOOKS

## Trusted • Reliable • Certified

- 40+ titles available
- Comply with accreditation and regulatory bodies
- Suitable for caregivers, boomers with elderly parents, health workers, auxiliary health staff & patients
- Self study style with "test yourself" section
- Health On the Net (HON) certified

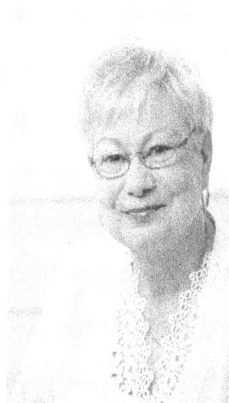

### Some of our titles:

| | | |
|---|---|---|
| Alzheimers Disease | Arthritis | Multiple Sclerosis |
| Pain | Strokes | Elder Abuse |
| Falls Prevention | Incontinence | Nutrition & Aging |
| Personal Care | Positioning | Confusion |
| Transferring people | Care of the Back | Skin Care |

For complete list of titles go to www.mediscript.net

Contact: 1 800 773 5088
Fax 1800 639 3186 • Email: mediscript30@yahoo.ca

# CONTENTS

# INTRODUCTION

This book provides basic, non controversial and trusted information that can help a wide spectrum of readers.

The primary objective of the information is to help a person provide effective quality care to a loved one or someone in his or her care.

Your role as a caregiver could mean the older person in your care is a family member or loved one, or you may be a non family member who is helping out a friend. Alternatively, you may be a paid health worker providing quality care for a client. With this in mind, we will alternate between referring to family members, loved ones, older persons and clients.

All the information is reliable and was written by a group of eminent nurse educators who ensured the information complies with best practice guidelines and satisfies the various accreditation and regulatory bodies. Because there is so much unreliable information on the internet, you can be assured the "All About" publications are HON (Health On the Net) certified.

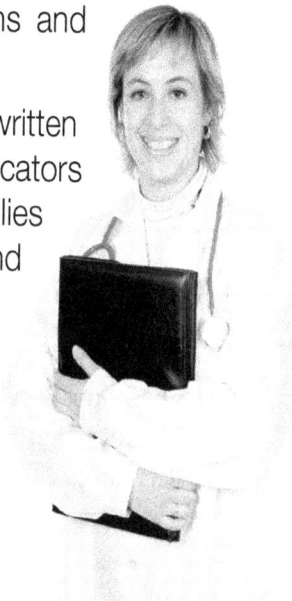

# AN IMPORTANT MESSAGE
# FROM THE PUBLISHER

Each person's treatment, advice, medical aids, physical therapy and other approaches to health care are unique and highly dependant upon the diagnosis and overall assessment by the medical team.

We emphasize therefore that the information within this book is not a substitute for the advice and treatment from a health care professional.

This book provides generic information concerning skin care for older people, the critical factors associated with skin care, and common sense well established skin care practices.

With all this in mind, the publishers and authors disclaim any responsibility for any adverse effects resulting directly or indirectly from the suggestions contained within this book or from any misunderstanding of the content on the part of the reader.

# HAVE YOU HEARD

## The following notices were found in various locations:

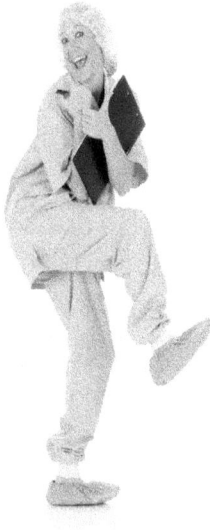

- **In the window of an Oregon store:** Why go elsewhere and be cheated, when you can come here.

- **In the window of a maternity clothes store:** We are open on labour day.

- **In a cemetery:** Persons are prohibited from picking flowers from any but their own graves.

- **On a highway:** When this sign is under water, this road is impassable.

- **On the door of a maternity ward:** Push Push Push

# HOW MUCH DO YOU KNOW

It helps to figure out how much you know before starting. In this way you will have an idea as to the gaps in your knowledge prior to reading the content. Please circle to indicate the best answer. Remember, at this stage, you are not expected to know all the answers:

**1.** What do you think is the worst skin problem?

a. Chronic wound

b. Skin tear

c. Ostomy

d. Psoriasis

**2.** What name below is NOT part of the skin anatomy?

a. Epidermis

b. Eccrine glands

c. Cartilage

d. Melanocyte

**3.** Which one of the following is NOT a known risk factor for developing skin problems?

a. Diabetes

b. Incontinence

c. Too much lotion

d. Excessive perspiration

**4.** Which of the following is NOT a function of the skin?

a. Vitamin production

b. Communication

c. Regulates optimum dryness

d. Passive barrier

**5.** Which of the following skin care products or practices should NOT be done?

a. Massage at risk areas to improve circulation.

b. Apply several applications of skin care lotion in one day.

c. Too frequent inspections of the skin.

d. Turning a patient at risk for pressure ulcers.

**6.** Which one of the following is NOT recommended to avoid damage of skin from the sun?

a. Avoid the sun from 10:00AM to 4:00PM.

b. Apply recommended sun screen as soon as you get into the sun.

c. Wear clothes that are dark and cover arms and legs.

d. Ideally wear a wide brimmed hat.

**7.** Which one of the following parts of the body is most vulnerable to serious skin damage?

a. Nose

b. Shoulders

c. Foot

d. Neck

# ANSWERS

**1.** a. Chronic wounds can take a long time to heal and greatly affect the quality of life of the patient. They can also incur great expense in terms of time on the part of the caregiver and health care professional and cost a lot in product purchases.

**2.** c. Cartilage is below the skin within the musculoskeletal system. Epidermis is the top layer of the skin, eccrine glands are sweat glands and melanocytes are the cells that provide the pigment melanin for skin color.

**3.** c. Too much lotion is not a known risk factor for developing skin problems. The nature of lotion is such that it evaporates quickly and it is usually recommended that lotions are applied frequently. Excessive perspiration and incontinence can macerate the skin, making it soft and vulnerable. Diabetes causes high blood sugar in the capillaries which can damage the nerve endings and blood circulation efficiency.

**4.** c. The skin does not regulate optimum dryness. It should always be hydrated and dryness should always be avoided.

**5.** a. Massaging at risk skin areas can do damage to the skin; placing direct heat towards the skin area can also be harmful. Excess lotion and frequent inspections can rarely do any harm. Careful turning of patients at risk for pressure ulcers is advocated to relieve excess pressure on at risk skin areas.

**6.** b. Apply recommended sun screen as soon as you get into the sun. It is highly recommended to apply 15 – 20 minutes before going outside.

**7.** c. The foot can have all sorts of problems, the main one being foot ulcers, chronic wounds caused by diabetes and skin damage.

---

### SOMETHING TO THINK ABOUT...

All would live long,

but none would be old.

Benjamin Franklin

---

## ABOUT THE SKIN

Skin consist of three different layers: the epidermis, dermis and fat and as we age the there is a natural thinning of the outer layer (epidermis) which leads to wrinkling and less protection and more vulnerability to injury due to this thinner skin.

Other factors such as heredity, environment, lifestyle, self care habits, detrimental risk factors and others collectively contribute to skin health.

When it comes to caring for the skin, an ounce of prevention is definitely worth a pound of cure.

The good news about prevention tactics for skin care in the elderly is that for the most part they are based on common sense, are usually non invasive and require simple vigilance and consistent maintenance.

---

### CONSIDER FOR A MOMENT...

The skin sheds and regrows outer skin cells every 27 days. By the age of 70, an average person will have shed 105 lbs. of skin cells.

---

# ANATOMY OF THE SKIN

The skin acts as a tough, self repairing, flexible covering without which we would fall apart. It protects us from the harmful rays of sunlight and any physical injury. If we get too hot, the skin enables sweating; our blood vessels dilate, changing our skin color to red, and this has the regulatory effect of cooling us down. The skin also keeps water out and, equally important, keeps our body fluids inside us.

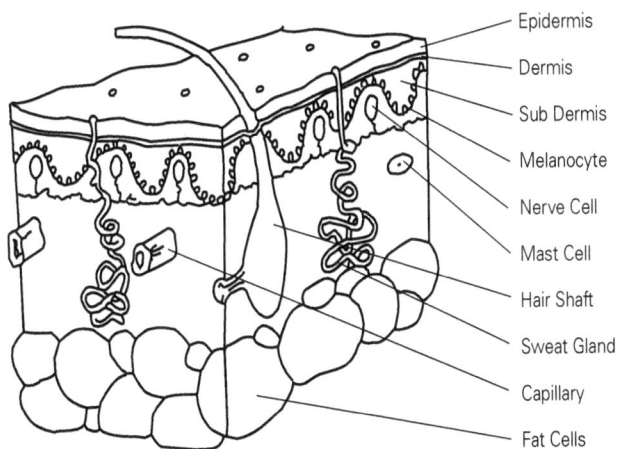

**Cross Section of Skin**

The skin has two distinct layers, the epidermis and the dermis. The epidermis is the layer nearest the surface and is about as thick as a piece of writing paper. There are no blood vessels or nerves in it, so if a pin is pushed sideways through this outer layer of skin, it will not bleed or hurt.

Most of the parts listed are self explanatory – the melanocytes provide the pigment for the skin.

The outer layer of the epidermis is constantly being replaced by new cells (approximately every 28 days). This outer layer is usually thin but for obvious reasons thicker on the palms and soles of the hands and feet.

The dermis and subdermis provide the support; further support, below the dermis and subdermis, is provided by fat.

There are two types of sweat glands: Eccrine, which produce watery sweat to cool the body, and Aprocrine, found in the groin and armpits, which contribute to body odor.

---

### SOMETHING TO THINK ABOUT...

The skin acts like an automatic air conditioner, maintaining the core body temperature of 98.6 degrees, while normal skin temperature is 92 degrees.

---

# FUNCTIONS OF SKIN

## Barrier

The skin acts as a passive barrier, protecting the body from the environment, and preventing damage from water, chemicals, bacteria, irradiation and direct injury from trauma. It also acts as a selective "dynamic" barrier to salts and heat.

## Regulates temperature

By way of its sensory components which communicate to the sweat glands, blood vessels and other skin parts, the skin ensures that the body is protected from extremes of temperature.

## Sensory functions

The skin can detect vibrations and temperature and relays this information to the various cells of the body to react accordingly.

## Communication functions

The skin has so many ways to communicate socially and sexually that we tend to take them for granted and perhaps not appreciate the innate and complex sophisticated qualities of this body organ.

### Water balance

Our bodies need to be optimally hydrated; the skin through its excretion glands and other functions ensures that optimum hydrations levels are maintained.

### Vitamin production

The skin also carries out some metabolic functions such assisting in the production of vitamin D.

---

**DID YOU KNOW**

Technically the sun is a carcinogen, because, just like smoking, it is a direct cause of cancer.

---

# CHANGES OF SKIN DUE TO AGING

## Fragile skin

There is a 1% decrease each year in the collagen levels in the dermis of the skin, causing a thinning of the outer layer of the skin (the epidermis and dermis). Collagen provides the skin's tensile strength so loss of it can contribute to wrinkling. Also, elastin fibers in the dermis of the skin provide the skin's elasticity. Loss of this elastin contributes to the skin's tendency to sag and wrinkle. See Fig. 2

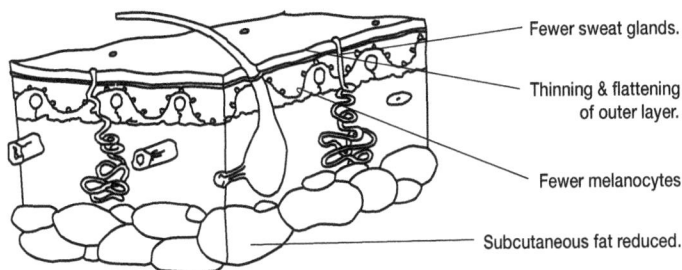

Fewer sweat glands.

Thinning & flattening of outer layer.

Fewer melanocytes

Subcutaneous fat reduced.

## Increased dryness of the skin

Over time, the eccrine glands decrease and the sweat glands produce less sweat. This collectively contributes to drier skin. Hydration of the skin is a fine balance for the elderly person; under- and over-hydration of the skin are fundamental causes of unhealthy skin.

## Less blood circulation

As the skin's dermis thins, fewer blood vessels are available leading to a decreased blood supply. This means there are fewer nutrients, oxygen and other components vital for the healing process being circulated within the body.

## Slowing epidermis cell replacement

Renewed cells are replaced at a slower rate which has implications for vital skin health and for any healing process that needs to take place.

## Sensory decline

Due to a variety of reasons such as nerve damage or loss and decreased blood circulation, there is a gradual decrease in sensation to pressure and light touch.

## Less immunity to infection

There is a loss of Langerhans cells which are responsible for the development of the bacteria-fighting defense mechanisms of the epidermis in order to counteract skin infections.

## Loss of hair and pigment of the skin

There is a decrease in the melanocytes (the pigment-producing cells) which can lead to the loss of melanin and cause graying of the hair and reduced hair growth.

## Loss of skin's full, healthy look

The subcutaneous fat on the hands, face, shins, waist (in men) and thighs (in women) tends to atrophy over time, leading to sagging and folds in the skin.

# RISK FACTORS FOR THE ELDERLY

Clearly the major risk factor contributing to the integrity of the skin is aging and subsequent fragile skin.

All of the following risk factors can contribute in their own way to skin damage but for the institutionalized elderly, the consequences of excess moisture on the skin through fecal or urinary incontinence or wound drainage are by far the biggest problems.

## Fragile skin

Usually as a result of the aging process on the skin, an overall fragility becomes an at risk characteristic of the elderly person. The outer layer, the epidermis, is only one cell thick but this becomes even thinner and provides less protection from physical injury and from hostile extrinsic factors such as bacteria. Less sweat gland production and fewer eccrine glands can contribute to much dryer skin, making it more prone to cracking and itching (scratching) which can damage the skin and even cause infection.

## What to do

- Make sure you protect the skin against any trauma such as banging into objects by way of making the environment as safe as possible (remove slippery rugs, do not excessively wax the floor, install grab bars in the bathroom, avoid furniture clutter, etc.).

• Ensure proper-fitting, breathable clothing to ensure comfort and unrestricted movement.

• Pad and protect any at-risk bony areas of the skin.

• Always "patch test" (try a little first to see if there is any skin reaction) a product before using, so as to avoid any traumatic allergy reaction.

• Avoid over bathing, excess heat and irritating lotions.

• Use pH-balanced soaps – remember, too, alkaline is caustic to the skin.

• Use humectant creams and lotions; they optimize moisture content for the skin.

## Incontinence (urine)

If urine comes into contact with the skin on a regular basis, there is a chance of chafing; in the elderly, however, this can progress to the more serious incontinence dermatitis condition. Urine comes into contact with skin which is often dry and cracked, providing an ideal environment for bacteria to grow which in turn produces ammonia on the skin and subsequently raises the pH of the skin. This in turn reduces the skin's defense mechanisms against bacteria, making it much more vulnerable to skin breakdown from a variety of causes.

## What to do

- The use of modern underpads that absorb moisture and present a quick drying surface with the skin can help and are preferable to products made of cloth.

- Use recommended moisture protectant creams and ointments.

- When petroleum or zinc based protectant products are used, they must be removed and reapplied following each incontinent episode. You have to be careful here of the danger of causing more skin damage due to the friction of removing these products.

- Try to ensure regular visits to the toilet.

- Find out the reason for the incontinence and the type of incontinence which may help in managing the situation.

- Medication can sometimes control certain types of incontinence.

- Address the issue of odour control through the use of underwear or whatever the health care professional recommends.

## Incontinence (fecal)

This problem offers greater medical concern because as feces pass through the gastrointestinal tract, digestive enzymes are deactivated. When feces mix with urine on the skin, the urine converts to ammonia, and the resultant alkaline pH activates the digestive enzymes, further increasing the risk of skin breakdown and bacterial infection.

### What to do

- Try to ensure fecal containment.

- Take measures for odor control.

- Apply protectant barrier creams or ointment to maintain the integrity of your skin.

- Try to establish regular bowel habits.

- Increase bulk and fiber into meals.


## Periwound maceration (skin area around the wound becoming soft)

The skin around a wound area such as a pressure or venous ulcer can be damaged by excess wound drainage or moisture. Wound exudate contains not only water, which can be detrimental, but also cellular debris and enzymes which can be additionally corrosive to the intact skin surrounding the wound.

Another negative factor can be dressings which leak and are only changed after the leakage has occurred; as a result the surrounding skin is exposed to potentially damaging wound exudates on a sustained basis. This moisture and maceration can increase the skin's permeability to irritating substances, increasing the possibility for infection, delayed healing time, and enlargement of the wound.

### What to do

- Traditionally, zinc oxide or petroleum is used as a protective barrier – this is usually effective in preventing contact of the wound exudates with the periwound skin area. You will have to be aware that these products can be messy and sometimes difficult to remove. They can also interfere with the dressing's absorption and adhesion.

- Also, consider other more modern skin barrier products, such as liquid-forming barrier films. These are easy to apply, conformable, resist being washed off, have low sensitization rates and do not trap containments.

- A change of dressing may contain the exudates more effectively.

## Skin adhesive products causing damage

Tapes, adhesive bandages and dressings such as hydrocolloids, films and some foams that strip the skin also may compromise the skin's barrier properties. Skin adhesion between products and skin varies. High adhesion products can have a bonding pressure that can cause skin tears if inappropriately removed.

### What to do

Acrylic adhesives, primarily found in film dressings, are best removed by pulling bilaterally to decrease the skin bond before lifting off the skin.

Spend a bit more time, being as careful as possible, when removing a skin adhesive product from the skin.

- Check with an expert to find out the best technique for removing a particular skin adhesive product.

### Pressure points on the bony prominences of the skin

Skin damage can occur where the skin is thinnest and over a bony area, such as the heels, lower back, elbows or shoulders.

When the person is immobilized and body movements are restricted, the weight of the body no longer has the opportunity to shift from one position to another, as it will normally do during sleep. The soft tissue or skin trapped between the bed and the bony prominences is compressed under the weight of the body and capillary blood flow is reduced or completely cut off. The skin damage that can result from this situation is called a pressure ulcer.

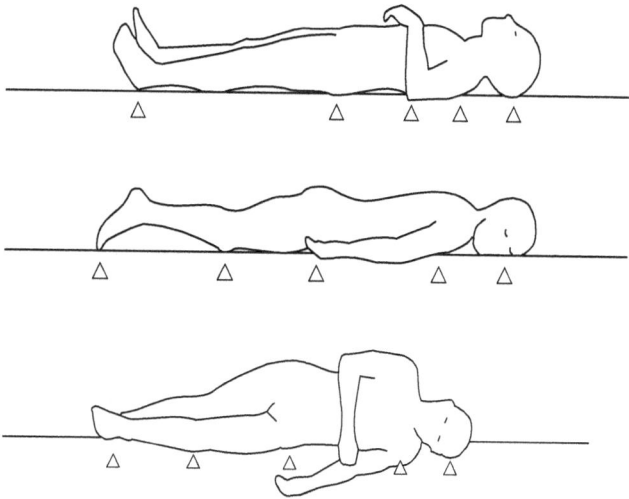

## What to do

- Be vigilant and look for early warning signs around bony prominences. Watch for pink, red or mottled unbroken skin that stays that way 20 minutes after the pressure is relieved.

- For an immobile client, turn the patient or shift positions every 2 hours.

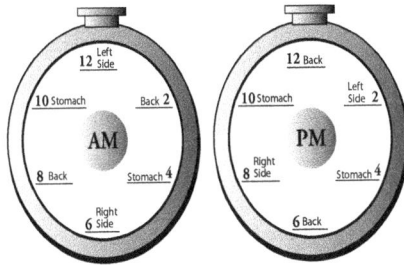

AM clock: 12 Left Side, 10 Stomach, 8 Back, 6 Right Side, 4 Stomach, 2 Back

PM clock: 12 Back, 10 Stomach, 8 Right Side, 6 Back, 4 Stomach, 2 Left Side

- Make sure any pressure relieving device, such as a special bed, boot, mattress etc., is being used properly.

- Follow the skin care program recommended by your health care professional.

- If a pressure ulcer exists, ensure the dressing is changed regularly and maintain proper hygiene procedures.

- Do not massage over the bony prominences; there is more risk of damage than improving blood circulation.

- Adhere to a sound nutrition plan and any recommended exercise/activity programs.

### Decreased mobility

People at risk for skin damage due to immobility include: bedridden patients; people who use wheelchairs; people with

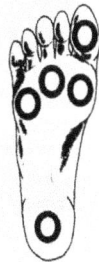

severe or chronic injuries, especially spinal cord injuries, and unconscious, post surgical (temporarily at high risk) or lethargic patients.

## What to do

- Exercise the client's joints and muscles regularly to relieve pressure and stimulate circulation.

- If possible, get the person out of bed as often as possible.

- Change the person's position in the wheelchair or chair every half hour, making sure to reposition the coccyx (tailbone) and hip pressure points.

- Make sure you have an adequate supply of pillows, towels and protective devices as appropriate to protect high risk areas. Heel protectors are a highly effective aid in preventing these problems.

- Ensure the client's feet do not rest directly against an unpadded footboard.

- Make sure the client is comfortable after turning or repositioning.

- If the patient is bedridden, change the position every two hours

## Diabetes

This is a major risk factor for the elderly due to the danger of developing diabetic foot ulcers. These are usually slow to heal and greatly affect one's quality of life. Diabetes causes high blood sugar which in turn causes nerve damage in the feet and reduced blood circulation to the surface of the foot. This dual combination contributes to the development of ulcers on the pressure points of the foot as shown below. The major reason for developing foot ulcers is mostly due to the lack of feeling in the foot, commonly known as the insensate foot. In such a case, an object may become lodged in a patient's foot/shoe, and because the patient cannot feel the sensation of pain, the object can damage the foot. Because there is an inadequate supply of blood to the foot, the ulcer can take a long time to heal.

## What to do

- Look for danger signs of a foot ulcer developing.
- Make sure glucose monitoring is taking place and that the diet, exercise, medication or insulin is being adhered to.
- Practice foot care through thorough inspection, daily wash and dry, skin care recommendations, toe nail care, recommended shoes and socks and walking tips.

## Shearing forces

A person confined to a bed, sliding slowly downwards from the sitting position, causes the skin to be pulled or stretched, interrupting the blood supply to the skin. Excessive shearing can affect deeper tissues; friction can cause the surface of the skin to be rubbed away faster than it can be replaced.

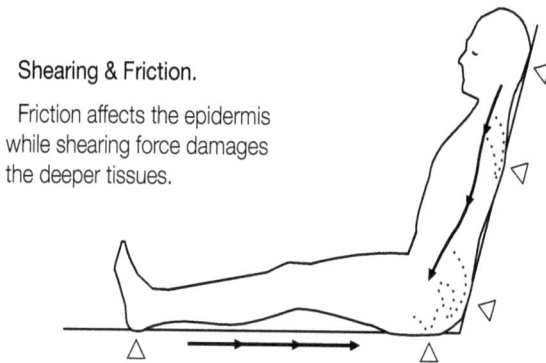

**Shearing & Friction.**

Friction affects the epidermis while shearing force damages the deeper tissues.

## What to do

- When in bed the person's head should be only slightly elevated to spread the body weight over a wider surface area and prevent sliding downward in the bed.

- Take care to follow procedures for correctly transferring patients or moving within the bed.

## Friction

This is created when skin and sheets or bedclothes rub together. This may happen when:

A person is pulled across rough or wrinkled sheets;

Food crumbs have not been removed, or

Skin rubs against a body brace or traction device.

### What to do

- Maintain the patient's bed so that the sheets are a possible source of friction.

- Eliminate all food crumbs and other objects such as pens, cards, etc. on the bed to avoid the unnoticed possibility of friction or pressure occurring.

- Keep the area around the bed as tidy as possible with bedside space to place objects away from the bed.

### Other factors

Smoking, malnutrition, swelling are just a few but review the following checklist page of all the risk factors:

# CHECKLIST FOR RISK

Name _____

| | | | |
|---|---|---|---|
| Fragile skin | ❏ | Incontinence | ❏ |
| Too much sun | ❏ | Circulation problems | ❏ |
| Perspiration | ❏ | Pressure points | ❏ |
| Shearing forces | ❏ | Dermatitis | ❏ |
| Friction | ❏ | Edema (swelling) | ❏ |
| Poor hygiene | ❏ | Infection | ❏ |
| Decreased mobility | ❏ | Skin adhesives | ❏ |
| Emaciation | ❏ | Diabetes | ❏ |
| Mental confusion | ❏ | Decreased sensation | ❏ |
| Foot care | ❏ | Wound seepage | ❏ |
| Poor nutrition | ❏ | Maceration | ❏ |
| Smoking | ❏ | Fistula drainage | ❏ |
| Obesity | ❏ | Stoma drainage | ❏ |

Tick any risk factor you think needs addressing.

# SKIN CARE PRODUCTS

There are many categories of skin care products on the market which are essentially developed to help maintain skin integrity or manage or treat common dermatological conditions such as dry skin and fungal infections. Many of these specifically address what is called the periwound skin (the immediate area around the wound) but it is important to note that they are not indicated for use in open wounds.

The categories of products you may come across include: cleansing products, moisture barriers and powders, moisturizers, sealants and protectants, tape, antimicrobials or antifungal preparations and topical anti-inflammatory and antipruritic (anti-itching) preparations.

To further increase the number of options, these products can come in tubes, jars, bottles, foam applicators, spray pumps, gels, ointments, wipes, creams, pastes, powders, and swabs. There are also fluid container products such as dressings, briefs or underpads.

Always follow the recommendations of your health care professional or facility to ensure the optimum products for the situation.

Skin care products are usually broken down into two basic categories:

Physical **barriers** are defined as a permanent interface between two surfaces to protect skin integrity.

**Protectants** are defined as indirect temporary techniques or applications to maintain the integrity of skin at high risk.

*Physical barrier skin products*

## Zinc oxide preparations

These are the most widely used barrier preparations and have been used for a long time and have been used routinely to protect the periwound skin. In babies, for diaper rash and people with sensitive skin, including the elderly, these zinc oxide and petroleum based skin barrier products have proven to be very helpful.

These products are stiff in texture, easily accessible and inexpensive, making them conducive for general use and the most part generally effective. There is significant product variability between preparations especially with regard to stiffness; sometimes ingredients such as perfumes can be allergenic which can in turn be detrimental to the skin.

Although inexpensive, you have to consider that the application of these products is labour-intensive and there is sometimes a danger of bacterial contamination.

Further, due to their stiff texture they can clog containment devices and interfere with absorbency, adhesion and antimicrobial properties of topical treatments. They are often messy and difficult to remove.

A further significant problem for the caregiver is that the underlying skin can be "masked" and not easy to assess.

## Adhesive dressings

Films or thin hydrocolloid dressings are also used as skin barriers. They are applied using a picture window framing technique, where a hole is cut in the dressing to allow for the movement of effluent into a management device such as an absorbent dressing, while protecting the skin around the wound margin. Framing the surrounding skin prevents effluent from attacking healthy skin by forming a solid interface between the two components.

This approach has the benefit of providing a constant barrier that does not require frequent changing (providing more comfort) but allows visualization of the underlying skin through the dressing. However, it must be pointed out that skills are needed by the caregiver/health professional to choose the optimum "draining" aperture.

There can be some disadvantages in that the dressing edge rolls or lifts, trapping the exudates and perhaps leading to the growth of bacteria. Hydrocolloid dressings can contribute to a developing odor which can cause problems and there is always a possibility of an allergic reaction.

### Liquid forming barriers

These products are relatively new, require skill to use but providing some important user benefits, such as: they are user-friendly, flexible, conformable and easy-to-use, allow uniform application, resist wash off, do not trap containments and you can see the underlying skin.

### Protectant skin products

### Skin cleansers or cleansing regimens

These products, which are known as surfactants, meaning they lower the surface tension, are designed to remove debris from the skin surface. They should not be used for open wounds where they can have a detrimental effect on healing.

Skin cleansers are characteristically mild, non-irritating and non-drying and are available in a wide variety of forms such as wipes, swabs, foams, washcloths, and bottles. They can be used in the bath, locally or in the shower.

There are more specialized periwound cleansers which gently dissolve and remove feces and urine, without having to scrub which could create more damage to the skin. They are also soapless and non-irritating.

It is always important to check that the right product is being used – there are further category variables such as sterile or non-sterile, ionic and non-ionic, and some are more toxic than others. Overuse can cause problems such as drying the skin and adversely changing the skin pH. There can also be sensitizers present.

## Moisturizers

These products are vital to ensure healthy skin maintenance and must be applied regularly.

The top layer of the skin needs 10% moisture content to maintain integrity. As previously described in skin structure, the very top layer of skin is the epidermis (next to the deeper, thicker dermis). It is this horny layer (stratum corneum) that provides protection from water loss. This is the layer of skin that must be kept supple and moist to ensure its integrity and this is where moisturizers can help.

You should evaluate whether the environment can be a risk factor; for example, warm climates or even an above average room temperature can deplete the body of protective moisture.

A further consideration is to ensure the moisturizer is applied to intact skin, otherwise there may be a sensation of stinging or burning.

Moisturizers, which usually consist of urea or lactic acid preparations, act as hydrators or lubricants. They act by binding moisture within the skin and their function is to preserve the suppleness of the skin and also act as a protection against harmful factors.

## GUIDE TO MOISTURIZERS

| Effective | More Effective | Very Effective |
|---|---|---|
| Lotions | Creams | Ointments |
| Consists of 90% or more water containing dissolved crystals held in suspension by surfactants. On application, feels cool, but evaporates quickly and must be applied frequently. | Consists of oil and water which is more occlusive than lotions and work more by preventing moisture loss due to evaporation rather than replenishing skin moisture. Creams need only to be applied 3- 4 times a day. | Consist of oil (usually lanolin or petroleum) and water in a proportion that has more occlusive properties ensuring a longer lasting form of moisturizer. They need much less applications than lotions or creams. |

## Fluid managers

These are absorbent devices that remove fluids from the skin surface, the common ones being diapers/ underpads and dressings.

There are many different categories of dressings and although absorbency may be a common feature, each type of dressing absorbs differently. An alginate dressing, for example, has the ability to absorb a huge amount of fluid whereas others just wick away fluid from the skin and soon create a seepage situation where fluid is leaking from the dressing. Other dressings provide a dynamic equilibrium on the wound surface. In any event, fluid leaking from dressings causing "strike through" can damage the skin.

Diapers or underpads vary a great deal in functional qualities. You should be aware of the recommended products available from your facility or provider and follow the instructions.

Ostomy bags are another example of a fluid container. These are pouches attached to patients to relieve excretion after intestinal surgery. While the health care provider has the expertise in this area and is responsible for selection of the relevant product, patient education and training is vital.

## OTHER SKIN CARE PRODUCTS

Although protectants and moisturizers make up most of the numerous skin care products, here are some others you may come across:

### Antimicrobial/antifungal preparations

These are available as creams, pastes and powders, both over the counter and with prescription to treat bacterial or fungal infections.

### Mucosal care products

These are used for the cleaning and care of mucosal membranes and oral lesions.

### Perineal cleansers

Although these are technically cleansers and in the category of moisturizers, they deserve a special mention because there are a lot of brands in this category. There is a great demand for these products for the elderly because of factors such as incontinence and wound care issues.

### Sealants

These specialized products are available as sprays, gels, ointments and wipes and are sometimes used on irritated skin or burns. It is very important to read and understand the instructions and indications for use before applying these products to irritated or broken skin.

# COMMON SKIN CONDITIONS
# OF THE ELDERLY

The following conditions require a health care professional's attention and treatment but it advisable for you to be aware of them and practical advice is given in other "all about" books such as "wound Care Principles".

## Skin Tears

This is a separation or peeling back of the outer layer (epidermis) of the skin, usually occurring on the upper body.

## Senile Purpura

This means easy bruising of the skin  due to the skin becoming thinner.

## Xerosis (Aeteatotic Eczema)

This is a worsening of already dry skin due to decreasing oil content and causes increased itching.

## Blistering disorders

There can be different causes such as viruses (e.g. chicken pox reactivation), and immune disorders.

## Stasis dermatitis

This condition causes rashes around the ankles due to poor blood circulation with other symptoms such as redness, swelling and dry scaly skin. This could a precursor to a skin (venous) ulcer.

## Skin Cancer

Not all skin lumps or pigment changes are cancerous but it is important to have these observations checked out.

## Chronic wounds

These are skin ulcers caused by an underlying problem such as diabetes, poor blood circulation, fragile skin, prolonged pressure on vulnerable skin and so on. There is a lot you can do to prevent and help heal these wounds. More information is available on *All About Wound Care Principles*.

# EMOTIONAL ASPECTS OF SKIN CARE

From the perception of the elderly, quality of life issues are rated as follows:

**Independence:** Older people prefer NOT to rely on others for their basic functions

**Dignity:** Older people need to feel respected and controlling problems like incontinence or flaky skin can help keep the motivation for self care.

**Security:** Older people require a safe environment, free of financial worries can provide mental well being to ensure self help and self care habits.

**Pain:** Older people can cope better if any associated pain due to skin problems are addressed.

Consequently, appreciating the elderly person's perception is the reality; you should always practice a relationship that asks questions, listens and discusses issues. Always asking yourself "what would I want in this situation?"

# EMOTIONAL ISSUES CHECKLIST

| Concerns | Contributing factors | Action required |
|---|---|---|
| Independence | Loss of control of functions | |
| | Loss of mobility | |
| | Loss of memory | |
| | Cognitive ability | |
| | Ability to bathe or shower | |
| Dignity | Incontinence embarrassment | |
| | Nobody listens | |
| | Bad odor embarrassment | |
| | Flaky skin | |
| | Ugly, blotchy skin | |
| | Feeling ignored | |
| | Feeling treated like a child | |
| | Slow healing wound | |
| | Poor hygiene | |
| Pain | Inadequate medication | |
| | Self help tips suggested | |
| | Compression treatment | |

| Patient Centered Concerns | Contributing factors | Action required |
|---|---|---|
| | Nobody knows it is happening | |
| | Fear of addiction | |
| | No pain assessment conducted | |
| Too many pills | Over-prescribing | |
| | Poor monitoring or review | |
| | Drug interactions | |
| Relationships | No family visits | |
| | Limited socializing | |
| Embarrassment | Incontinence odor | |
| | Obvious skin problems | |
| | Cognitive ability | |
| Feeling of support | | Clubs available |
| | Chats from staff | |
| | Social services contact | |
| Security | Money worries | |
| | Accident anxiety | |

# CASE EXAMPLE

Mr. B is 83 years old, still active, with good cognitive ability, cooperative and is a good walker.

Lately his skin, especially on his legs, has become extremely dry and itchy and has recently broken the skin through scratching. His lower legs show some swelling and red staining marks around the ankle. His nurse had recently ordered compression stockings for him but he does not always use them because he finds them difficult to put on because of a chronic bad back.

*What would you do to help Mr. B?*

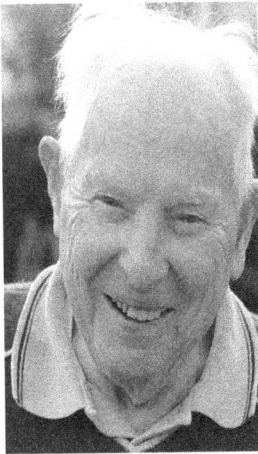

# YOUR ANSWERS TO CASE EXAMPLE

## SUGGESTED ANSWERS TO CASE EXAMPLE

Clearly you have the advantage here of a cooperative, motivated person who can help himself with some encouragement, explanations and the use of correct products.

The first thing to do is to prevent further scratching and treat the dry skin in line with the skin care products you have available. A soothing moisturizer is needed and any practical suggestions and encouragement to ensure Mr. B avoids actual scratching of the skin.

As compression stockings have been recommended and the symptoms of swelling, red stains indicate venous disease, Mr. B is at risk for developing a venous leg ulcer.

You must motivate and train him to put on his compression stockings everyday and overcome the bad back issue as a hindrance in putting on the stockings. If you sense a fitting or other technical problem, then you should inform the nurse.

# CONCLUSION

Providing and maintaining proper skin care in the elderly involves many activities, products and quality care practices adherence.

You cannot do much about the aging process but you can provide quality care and an optimum environment. For example, the Agency for Healthcare Research and Quality (AHRQ) suggests that low humidity (below 40%) and cool air can exacerbate dry skin, this is something you can control.

Care in transferring and positioning people, the use of protective padding and the diligent use of recommended skin care products are very important.

It is always preferable to prevent a medical condition from occurring in the first place. You should refresh yourself on these principles and be vigilant to try to prevent diabetic, venous, pressure or arterial skin ulcers. These usually become chronic wounds and can take a long time to heal.

Finally, skin care has to be regarded as team effort, the most important member of the team being the elderly person. It is pivotal to ensure the person knows she is part of the team, feels comfortable voicing her concerns and feelings, and is involved in the decision making process.

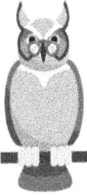

## CHECK YOUR KNOWLEDGE

1. Apart from the sun's UV rays and aging, name another risk factor.

2. Name one type of generic skin protectant product.

3. Name one example of a fluid manager type product.

4. Apart from fragile skin, name another change of the skin due to aging.

5. Name one common chronic wound that every effort should be made to prevent occurring.

# TEST YOURSELF

**1.** The components in the skin that deliver oxygen and nutrients to skin cells are:

a. Melanocytes

b. Capillaries

c. Eccrine glands

d. Dermis

**2.** The outermost layer of the skin is called :

a. Fat cells

b. Stratum corneum

c. Epidermis

d. Collagen

**3.** Which of the following best describes the functions of the skin?

a. Sensory perception, temperature regulation and protection

b. Skeletal support, sensation and communication

c. Protection, aging inhibitor, sweating

d. Nourishment, water balance and cooling

**4.** Which of the following is NOT a risk factor for poor skin integrity?

a. Diabetes

b. Decreased mobility of the client

c. Alginate dressings

d. Incontinence

**5.** Which of the following skin care products do you have to apply most frequently?

a. Creams

b. Ointments

c. Antimicrobials

d. Lotions

**6.** What percentage of moisture content does the top layer of skin need to maintain skin integrity?

a. 2%

b. 4%

c. 10%

d. 20%

**7.** Which of the following is NOT a common skin condition of the elderly?

a. Skin tear

b. Dry skin

c. Psoriasis

d. Senile purpura

# ANSWERS

1. b. Capillaries, the tiniest extensions of the blood circulatory system, release the necessary oxygen and nutrients into the skin cells. Eccrine glands are the sweat glands, melanocytes are the cells that produce melanin and the dermis is the second, thicker layer of the skin.

2. c. The epidermis is the one - cell, outermost layer of the skin, not to be confused with the dead skin layer above this which is called the stratum corneum.

3. a. Sensory perception, temperature regulation and protection are the three main vital functions of the skin. The other 3 options have marginal or incorrect components in the answer.

4. c. Alginate dressings have a high absorbency quality so the likelihood of seepage is minimal. Diabetes is a risk for foot ulcers, decreased mobility is a risk for pressure ulcers, and incontinence causes maceration and loss of skin integrity.

5. d. Lotions evaporate quickly because of the high water content and must be applied more frequently than the other products listed.

6. c. 10% is recognized as the approximate optimum amount needed to maintain supple, healthy skin.

7. c. Psoriasis is a skin condition experienced by all age groups.

# REFERENCES

Allman, R.M., Laprade, C.A., Noel, L.B., et al. Pressure sores among hospitalised patients. Annals of Internal Medicine. 1986; 105:337-342.

Bryant, R., Wysocki, A. Skin. In: Bryant R, ed. Acute and Chronic Wounds: Nursing Management. St. Louis, Mo.: Mosby Year Book Inc.; 1992.

Fowler, E.M., Ouslander, J., Paper, J. Managing incontinence in the nursing home population. J Enterostomal Ther. 1990; (17):77-86.

Kemp, M.G. Protecting the skin from moisture and associated irritants. J Gerontol Nurs. 1994; 20(9):8.

Phillips, T.J. OW/M commentary: a clinician's guide to common dermatological problems. Ostomy/Wound Management. 1994; 40(9):70-79.

Price, P. Health-related quality of life and the patient's perspective. Journal of Wound Care. 1998; 7(7):365-366.

Sams, W.M. Structure and function of the skin. In: Sams, W.M., Lynch, P.J., eds. Principles and Practice of Dermatology. New York, NY: Churchill Livingstone; 1990.

Sibbald, G., Cameron, J. Dermatological aspects of wound care. In: Krasner, D., Rodeheaver, G., Sibbald, R.G., eds. Chronic Wound Care: A Clinical Source Book for Healthcare Professionals, 3rd ed. Wayne, Pa: HMP Communications; 2001:275.

Sibbald, R.G., Campbell, K., Coutts, P., Queen, D. Intact skin – an integrity not to be lost. (2008). Retrieved January 7, 2011, from: http://www.o-wm.com/article/1757

Silverberg, N., Silverberg, L. Aging and the skin. Postgrad Med. 1989; 86:131. www.worldwidewounds.com"